AF885227

T3 EMT CASES WORKBOOK

TABLE OF CONTENTS

Introduction

1. Pediatric Anaphylaxis 1

2. Chest Pain 11

3. Respiratory – COPD 21

4. Stroke 31

5. Diabetic Emergency 41

6. Normal Delivery 51

7. Overdose- Narcotic 61

8. Schizophrenia 71

9. Blunt Head Injury 79

10. Heat Emergency 91

11. Partial Amputation 101

12. Soft Tissue – Burns 111

Appendix PCR Sheets 121

Introduction

Preparing to be an EMT is an arduous but rewarding journey. As you progress on this journey you will develop both psychomotor skills and as importantly critical thinking and reasoning abilities to reinforce the skills. The T3 Scenario cases are designed to provide an interactive classroom experience where you are in the heart of the action on simulated calls. As the cases unfold you will be called upon to make decisions and recall important information from your study. Going through the cases will tie concepts together for you.

Workbook Organization

Each chapter in this text corresponds to one of the T3 video cases. There are approximately 15-20 questions per case that cover knowledge, skills and affect. After every case you will find 2 PCR sheets for that case. These are designed for you to practice your documentation skills and also to help you deliver a good report of the call to medical control or handoff at the hospital.

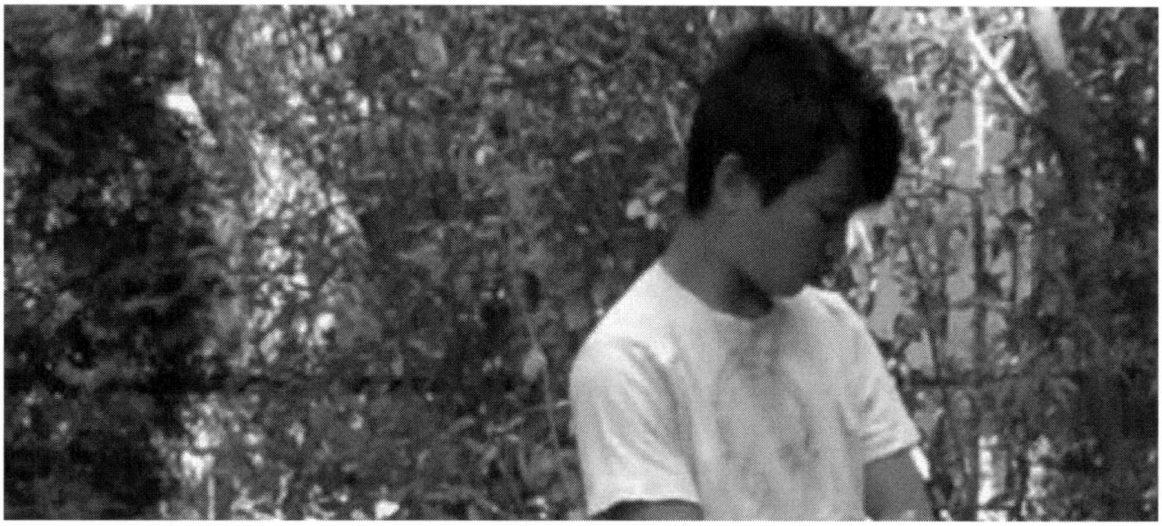

1 16 Y/O MALE, SHORTNESS OF BREATH AFTER BEE STING

DISPATCH

Location: Suburban backward

Type of situation: SOB after bee sting

Number of patients: 1

Hazards: No hazards

OBJECTIVES

1. Understand the pathophysiology of anaphylactic shock in pediatric patient.
2. Quickly assess and recognize anaphylaxis in pediatric patient.
3. Prioritize treatment for anaphylactic shock.
4. Appropriately manage patient's airway.
5. Exhibit teamwork and communication to evaluate and treat severe respiratory distress in children.

SCENE SIZE-UP	
OVERALL SAFETY	SCENE IS SAFE
MOI / NOI	SOB, BEE STING
RESOURCES	BLS RESPONSE
C-SPINE	NO SIGNS OF TRAUMA

ANAPHYLAXIS

QUESTIONS

Pause 1

Knowledge 0.35

WHAT COULD BE CAUSING THE DIFFICULTY BREATHING?

HOW WILL YOU DETERMINE THE SERIOUSNESS?

Pause 2

Communication 1.16

DISCUSS COMMUNICATION STRATEGIES WITH A PEDIATRIC PATIENT.

Pause 3

Assessment 1.52

WHAT IS SIGNIFICANT ABOUT PATIENTS SIGNS AND SYMPTOMS?

Pause 4

Knowledge 2.11

WHAT ARE YOUR ASSESSMENT PRIORITIES WITH THIS PATIENT?

QUESTIONS

Pause 5

Knowledge 2.58

HOW SERIOUS IS THIS PATIENT AND WHY?

Pause 6

Knowledge 3.05

HOW WILL YOU TREAT THIS PATIENT?

Pause 7

Communication 3.19

HOW CAN YOU HELP MANAGE THIS PATIENT'S ANXIETY?

Pause 8

Skill 3.25

WHAT ARE THE STEPS IN DRAWING UP THE EPINEPHRINE IF NO AUTO-INJECTOR IS AVAILABLE?

HOW WILL YOU PERFORM INTRAMUSCULAR INJECTION?

Pause 9

Assessment 4.35

WHAT IS IMPORTANT TO MONITOR WITH THE PATIENT NOW?

Pause 10

Transport 5.02

WHERE SHOULD PATIENT BE TRANSPORTED?

QUESTIONS

Pause 11

ALS INTERVENTIONS 5.15

Pause 12

Assessment 6.20

WHAT IS SIGNIFICANT ABOUT THE PATIENT"S VITALS?

WHAT DETERIORATION IS POSSIBLE AND HOW CAN IT BE MANAGED?

Pause 13

Skill 6.55

WHAT ARE SOME COMMON BVM PITFALL?

Pause 14

Communication 6.46

WHY IS THE MEDIC CALLING MEDICAL CONTROL?

Pause 15

Communication 8.41

WHAT INFORMATION IS IMPORTANT TO CONVEY IN YOUR RADIO REPORT AND PCR?

REFLECTION

WOULD YOU HAVE DONE ANYTHING DIFFERENTLY FROM THE ACTIONS AND DECISIONS SHOWN IN THE VIDEO ?

CRITIQUE THE PERFORMANCE AND EXPLAIN YOUR THOUGHT PROCESS.

EMS PATIENT CARE REPORT (PCR) Scenario:

PATIENT INFORMATION

Name:	Allergies:
Age:	Medications:
Sex:	Past Medical History:
Weight: Kg (lb)	Chief Complaint:

VITAL SIGNS

Time:	BP:	Pulse:	Respiration:	Sao_2:
Time:	BP:	Pulse:	Respiration:	Sao_2:
Time:	BP:	Pulse:	Respiration:	Sao_2:

PHYSICAL / NEUROLOGICAL EXAM

LOC:	Skin:	AB/GI:
Oriented:	HEENT:	Pelvis:
GCS:	Neck:	GU:
Pupils:	Chest:	Posterior :
Sensory/Motor:	Respiratory:	Extremities:
Facial Droop:	Cardiovascular:	Psychiatric:
Speech:	EKG:	GLU:

CHIEF COMPLAINT

HISTORY OF PRESENT ILLNESS

NOTES

EMS PATIENT CARE REPORT (PCR) Scenario:

PATIENT INFORMATION

Name:	Allergies:
Age:	Medications:
Sex:	Past Medical History:
Weight: Kg (lb)	Chief Complaint:

VITAL SIGNS

Time:	BP:	Pulse:	Respiration:	Sao_2:
Time:	BP:	Pulse:	Respiration:	Sao_2:
Time:	BP:	Pulse:	Respiration:	Sao_2:

PHYSICAL / NEUROLOGICAL EXAM

LOC:	Skin:	AB/GI:
Oriented:	HEENT:	Pelvis:
GCS:	Neck:	GU:
Pupils:	Chest:	Posterior :
Sensory/Motor:	Respiratory:	Extremities:
Facial Droop:	Cardiovascular:	Psychiatric:
Speech:	EKG:	GLU:

CHIEF COMPLAINT

HISTORY OF PRESENT ILLNESS

NOTES

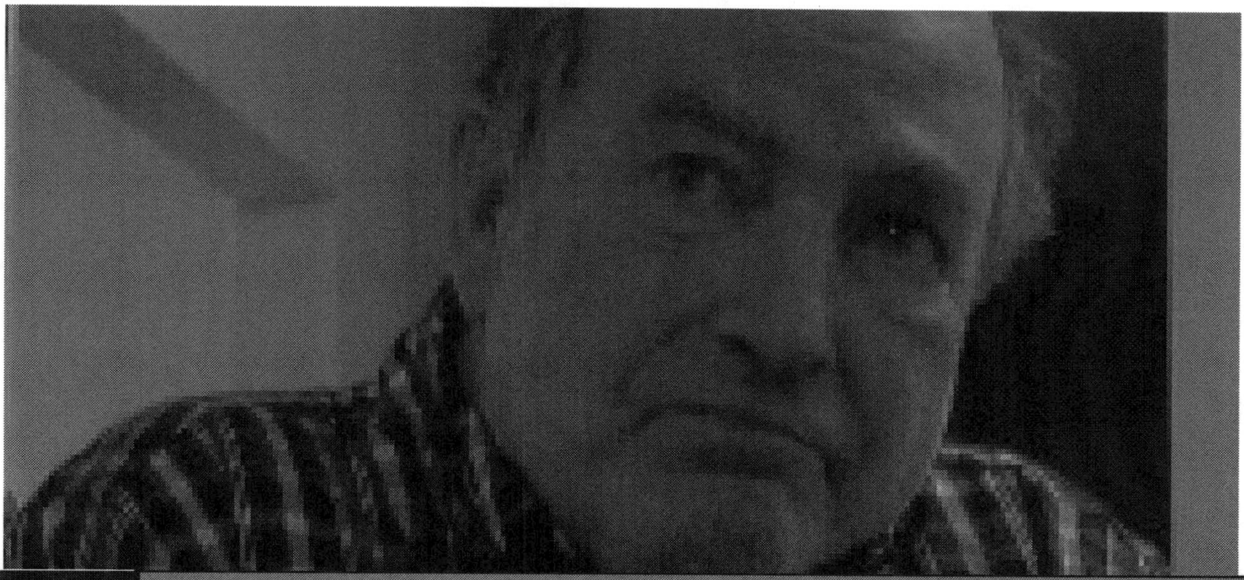

2 80 Y/O MALE, CHEST PAIN AND WEAKNESS

DISPATCH
Location: Apartment
Type of situation: Chest pain and weakness
Number of patients: 1
Hazards: No hazards

OBJECTIVES
1. Assessment of the scene and the patient.
2. Recognition of the signs and symptoms of cardiac compromise
3. Understand the pathophysiology of the cardiovascular system.
4. Explain the principles of CPR, AED use and resuscitation
5. Prioritization of interventions and treatment.
6. Teamwork, communication and division of duties

SCENE SIZE-UP	
OVERALL SAFETY	SCENE IS SAFE
MOI / NOI	CHEST PAIN AND WEAKNESS
RESOURCES	BLS RESPONSE
C-SPINE	NO SIGNS OF TRAUMA

CHEST PAIN

QUESTIONS

Pause 1

Knowledge 1.01

WHAT ARE POSSIBLE CAUSES OF CHEST PAIN IN THE ELDERLY?

Pause 2

Assessment 2.13

WHAT ARE POSSIBLE CAUSES OF GENERAL WEAKNESS INN THE ELDERLY?

Pause 3

Skill 2.19

WHAT WILL YOU INCLUDE IN YOUR PRIMARY ASSESSMENT FOR THIS PATIENT?

WHY IS THE PATIENT WEAK WHEN HE STANDS?

Pause 4

Skill 3.00

WHAT EFFECT WILL ASPIRIN HAVE HERE?

QUESTIONS

Pause 5

Assessment 3.23

WHAT ARE THE IMPORTANT ELEMENTS OF THE SECONDARY ASSESSMENT FOR THIS PATIENT?

Pause 6

Assessment 4.10

WHAT DO THE FINDINGS INDICATE?

WHAT ACTION WOULD YOU LIKE TO PERFORM NEXT?

Pause 7

Skill 5.05

WHAT IS THE SIGNIFICANCE OF VFIB RHYTHM ON MONITOR?

WHAT ACTIONS SHOULD BE PERFORMED WITH THE PATIENT IN THIS RHYTHM?

Pause 8

Skill 5.37

WHAT IS NEEDED FOR HIGH QUALITY CPR TO BE DELIVERED?

Pause 9

Knowledge 5.48

WHAT SHOULD HAPPEN AFTER 2 MINUTES OF CPR?

Pause 10

Knowledge 6.16

WHAT SEQUENCE OF EVENTS SHOULD TAKE PLACE NOW THAT PULSES HAVE RETURNED?

QUESTIONS

Pause 11

Reassessment and Transport 6.40

WHERE SHOULD THIS PATIENT BE TRANSPORTED?

WHAT ARE YOUR PRIORITIES IN THE AMBULANCE?

Pause 12

Communication 6.51

WHAT INFORMATION IS IMPORTANT TO CONVEY IN YOUR RADIO REPORT?

PCR

WHAT IS IMPORTANT TO DOCUMENT ON THIS PCR?

REFLECTION

WOULD YOU HAVE DONE ANYTHING DIFFERENTLY FROM THE ACTIONS AND DECISIONS SHOWN IN THE VIDEO ?

CRITIQUE THE PERFORMANCE AND EXPLAIN YOUR THOUGHT PROCESS.

EMS PATIENT CARE REPORT (PCR) Scenario:

PATIENT INFORMATION

Name:	Allergies:
Age:	Medications:
Sex:	Past Medical History:
Weight: Kg (lb)	Chief Complaint:

VITAL SIGNS

Time:	BP:	Pulse:	Respiration:	Sao_2:
Time:	BP:	Pulse:	Respiration:	Sao_2:
Time:	BP:	Pulse:	Respiration:	Sao_2:

PHYSICAL / NEUROLOGICAL EXAM

LOC:	Skin:	AB/GI:
Oriented:	HEENT:	Pelvis:
GCS:	Neck:	GU:
Pupils:	Chest:	Posterior :
Sensory/Motor:	Respiratory:	Extremities:
Facial Droop:	Cardiovascular:	Psychiatric:
Speech:	EKG:	GLU:

CHIEF COMPLAINT

HISTORY OF PRESENT ILLNESS

NOTES

EMS PATIENT CARE REPORT (PCR) Scenario:

PATIENT INFORMATION

Name:	Allergies:
Age:	Medications:
Sex:	Past Medical History:
Weight: Kg (lb)	Chief Complaint:

VITAL SIGNS

Time:	BP:	Pulse:	Respiration:	Sao_2:
Time:	BP:	Pulse:	Respiration:	Sao_2:
Time:	BP:	Pulse:	Respiration:	Sao_2:

PHYSICAL / NEUROLOGICAL EXAM

LOC:	Skin:	AB/GI:
Oriented:	HEENT:	Pelvis:
GCS:	Neck:	GU:
Pupils:	Chest:	Posterior :
Sensory/Motor:	Respiratory:	Extremities:
Facial Droop:	Cardiovascular:	Psychiatric:
Speech:	EKG:	GLU:

CHIEF COMPLAINT

HISTORY OF PRESENT ILLNESS

NOTES

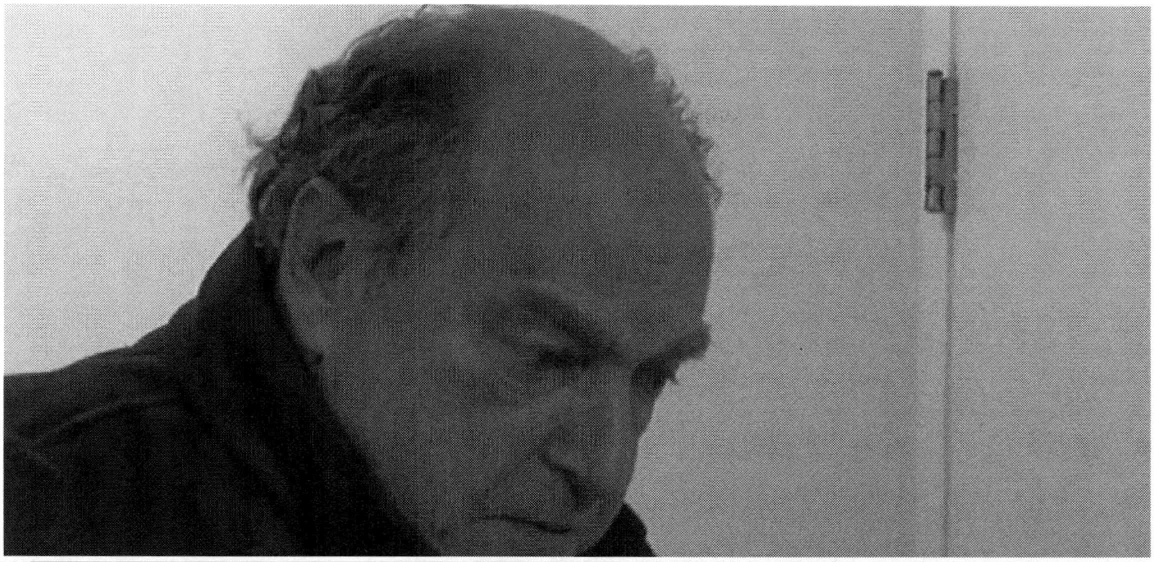

3 68 Y/O MALE, SHORTNESS OF BREATH

DISPATCH
Location: Suburban home
Type of situation:SOB, difficulty breathing
Number of patients: 1
Hazards: No hazards

OBJECTIVES

1. Assessment of the COPD patient
2. Understand the pathophysiology of COPD
3. Recognition of exacerbation of COPD
4. Prioritization and performance of interventions- O2, Nebulizer, CPAP
5. Recognition of exacerbation of COPD

SCENE SIZE-UP	
OVERALL SAFETY	SCENE IS SAFE
MOI / NOI	SHORTNESS OF BREATH
RESOURCES	ALS RESPONSE
C-SPINE	NO SIGNS OF TRAUMA

COPD

QUESTIONS

Pause 1

Knowledge 1.10

WHAT ARE POSSIBLE CAUSES OF RESPIRATORY DISTRESS IN THE ELDERLY ?

Pause 2

Assessment 2.05

IS THIS PATIENT SICK OR NOT SICK, WHY?

WHAT IS IMPORTANT TO ASSESS FOR THIS PATIENTS?

Pause 3

Knowledge 2.14

WHAT DO YOU WANT TO DO FIRST AND WHY?

Pause 4

Assessment 3.03

WHAT DO ASSESSMENT FINDINGS INDICATE?

WHAT ACTIONS SHOULD BE PERFORMED?

QUESTIONS

Pause 5

Skill 3.22

DESCRIBE THE STEPS INVOLVED IN ALBUTEROL ADMINISTRATION.

Pause 6

Assessment 4.22

IS ANYTHING SIGNIFICANT IN THE PATIENTS HISTORY?

Pause 7

Knowledge 4.59

HOW WOULD THE EMT TAKE OVER THE PATIENTS BREATHING?

WHAT ARE THE INDICATIONS AND CONTRAINDICATIONS FOR BVM USE?

Pause 8

Assessment 5.47

IS THE FACT THE PATIENT IS TIRED SIGNIFICANT?

Pause 9

Skill 5.55

DESCRIBE THE TECHNIQUE FOR CPAP APPLICATION.

Pause 10

ALS 6.22

QUESTIONS

Pause 11

Knowledge 7.08

WHAT ARE THE BENEFITS OF CAPNOGRAPHY FOR THIS PATIENT?

IS A CO2 READING OF 50 CAUSE FOR CONCERN?

Pause 12

Communication 8.10

WHAT INFORMATION IS IMPORTANT TO CONVEY IN YOUR RADIO REPORT?

PCR

WHAT IS IMPORTANT TO DOCUMENT ON THIS PCR?

REFLECTION

WOULD YOU HAVE DONE ANYTHING DIFFERENTLY FROM THE ACTIONS AND DECISIONS SHOWN IN THE VIDEO ?

CRITIQUE THE PERFORMANCE AND EXPLAIN YOUR THOUGHT PROCESS.

EMS PATIENT CARE REPORT (PCR) Scenario:

PATIENT INFORMATION

Name:	Allergies:
Age:	Medications:
Sex:	Past Medical History:
Weight: Kg (lb)	Chief Complaint:

VITAL SIGNS

Time:	BP:	Pulse:	Respiration:	Sao_2:
Time:	BP:	Pulse:	Respiration:	Sao_2:
Time:	BP:	Pulse:	Respiration:	Sao_2:

PHYSICAL / NEUROLOGICAL EXAM

LOC:	Skin:	AB/GI:
Oriented:	HEENT:	Pelvis:
GCS:	Neck:	GU:
Pupils:	Chest:	Posterior :
Sensory/Motor:	Respiratory:	Extremities:
Facial Droop:	Cardiovascular:	Psychiatric:
Speech:	EKG:	GLU:

CHIEF COMPLAINT

HISTORY OF PRESENT ILLNESS

NOTES

EMS PATIENT CARE REPORT (PCR) Scenario:

PATIENT INFORMATION

Name:	Allergies:
Age:	Medications:
Sex:	Past Medical History:
Weight: Kg (lb)	Chief Complaint:

VITAL SIGNS

Time:	BP:	Pulse:	Respiration:	Sao_2:
Time:	BP:	Pulse:	Respiration:	Sao_2:
Time:	BP:	Pulse:	Respiration:	Sao_2:

PHYSICAL / NEUROLOGICAL EXAM

LOC:	Skin:	AB/GI:
Oriented:	HEENT:	Pelvis:
GCS:	Neck:	GU:
Pupils:	Chest:	Posterior :
Sensory/Motor:	Respiratory:	Extremities:
Facial Droop:	Cardiovascular:	Psychiatric:
Speech:	EKG:	GLU:

CHIEF COMPLAINT

HISTORY OF PRESENT ILLNESS

NOTES

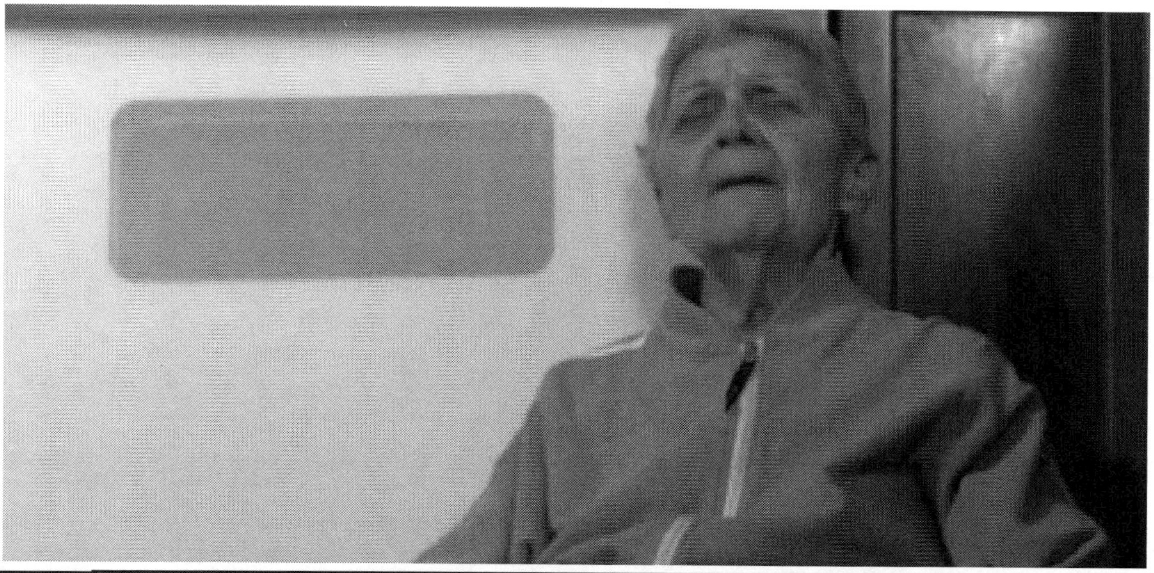

4 80 Y/O FEMALE, ALTERED MENTAL STATUS, POSSIBLE STROKE

DISPATCH
Location: Suburban home
Type of situation:AMS, possible stroke
Number of patients: 1
Hazards: No hazards

OBJECTIVES
1. Describe the Assessment and Treatment of a patient with a possible stroke
2. Demonstrate the use of a stroke assessment scale
3. Recognize other possible altered mental status causes
3. Prioritize and perform appropriate interventions.
5. Discuss the importance of transport destination and medical communication
6. Demonstrate effective teamwork

SCENE SIZE-UP	
OVERALL SAFETY	SCENE IS SAFE
MOI / NOI	ALTERED MENTAL STATUS, POSSIBLE STROKE
RESOURCES	ALS RESPONSE
C-SPINE	NO SIGNS OF TRAUMA

STROKE CASE

QUESTIONS

Pause 1

Knowledge 1.01

WHAT ARE POSSIBLE CAUSES OF ALTERED MENTAL STATUS?

WHAT ARE SIGNS AND SYMPTOMS ASSOCIATED WITH A STROKE PATIENT?

Pause 2

Assessment 1.59

WHAT CAN YOU GATHER FROM THIS NEW INFORMATION?

Pause 3

Resources 2.06

HOW WILL YOU AND YOUR PARTNER WORK TOGETHER FOR THIS PATIENT?

Pause 4

Assessment 2.16

WHAT DO YOU WANT TO DO FIRST AND WHY?

QUESTIONS

Pause 5

Communication 2.55

DISCUSS COMMUNICATION STRATEGIES WITH AN APHASIC PATIENT.

Pause 6

Stroke Scale 3.13

DESCRIBE HOW YOU WOULD USE A STROKE ASSESSMENT INSTRUMENT

Pause 7

Assessment 3.49

WHAT DO THE FINDINGS INDICATE?

Pause 8

Assessment4.10

WHAT DO THE VITALS INDICATE?

WHAT ARE THE TWO TYPES OF STROKE?

Pause 9

Assessment 4.22

IS THERE ANY ADDITIONAL INFORMATION YOU'D GATHER BEFORE LEAVING THE SCENE?

Pause 10

Transport 4.50

IS ANYTHING CONCERNING IN HER HISTORY?

WHERE SHOULD PATIENT BE TRANSPORTED?

QUESTIONS

Pause 11

Reassessment and Transport 5.15

WHAT ARE YOUR PRIORITIES IN THE AMBULANCE?

Pause 12

ALS INTERVENTIONS 6.11

In the ambulance the patient is placed on the monitor for a a 12 lead ECG to determine any cardiac conditions. The patient also has an IV started.

Pause 13

Communication 6.55

WHAT INFORMATION IS IMPORTANT TO CONVEY IN YOUR RADIO REPORT?

PCR

Documentation 7.47

WHAT IS IMPORTANT TO DOCUMENT ON THIS PCR?

REFLECTION

WOULD YOU HAVE DONE ANYTHING DIFFERENTLY FROM THE ACTIONS AND DECISIONS SHOWN IN THE VIDEO ?

CRITIQUE THE PERFORMANCE AND EXPLAIN YOUR THOUGHT PROCESS.

EMS PATIENT CARE REPORT (PCR) Scenario:

PATIENT INFORMATION

Name:	Allergies:
Age:	Medications:
Sex:	Past Medical History:
Weight: Kg (lb)	Chief Complaint:

VITAL SIGNS

Time:	BP:	Pulse:	Respiration:	Sao_2:
Time:	BP:	Pulse:	Respiration:	Sao_2:
Time:	BP:	Pulse:	Respiration:	Sao_2:

PHYSICAL / NEUROLOGICAL EXAM

LOC:	Skin:	AB/GI:
Oriented:	HEENT:	Pelvis:
GCS:	Neck:	GU:
Pupils:	Chest:	Posterior :
Sensory/Motor:	Respiratory:	Extremities:
Facial Droop:	Cardiovascular:	Psychiatric:
Speech:	EKG:	GLU:

CHIEF COMPLAINT

HISTORY OF PRESENT ILLNESS

NOTES

EMS PATIENT CARE REPORT (PCR) Scenario:

PATIENT INFORMATION

Name:	Allergies:
Age:	Medications:
Sex:	Past Medical History:
Weight: Kg (lb)	Chief Complaint:

VITAL SIGNS

Time:	BP:	Pulse:	Respiration:	Sao_2:
Time:	BP:	Pulse:	Respiration:	Sao_2:
Time:	BP:	Pulse:	Respiration:	Sao_2:

PHYSICAL / NEUROLOGICAL EXAM

LOC:	Skin:	AB/GI:
Oriented:	HEENT:	Pelvis:
GCS:	Neck:	GU:
Pupils:	Chest:	Posterior :
Sensory/Motor:	Respiratory:	Extremities:
Facial Droop:	Cardiovascular:	Psychiatric:
Speech:	EKG:	GLU:

CHIEF COMPLAINT

HISTORY OF PRESENT ILLNESS

NOTES

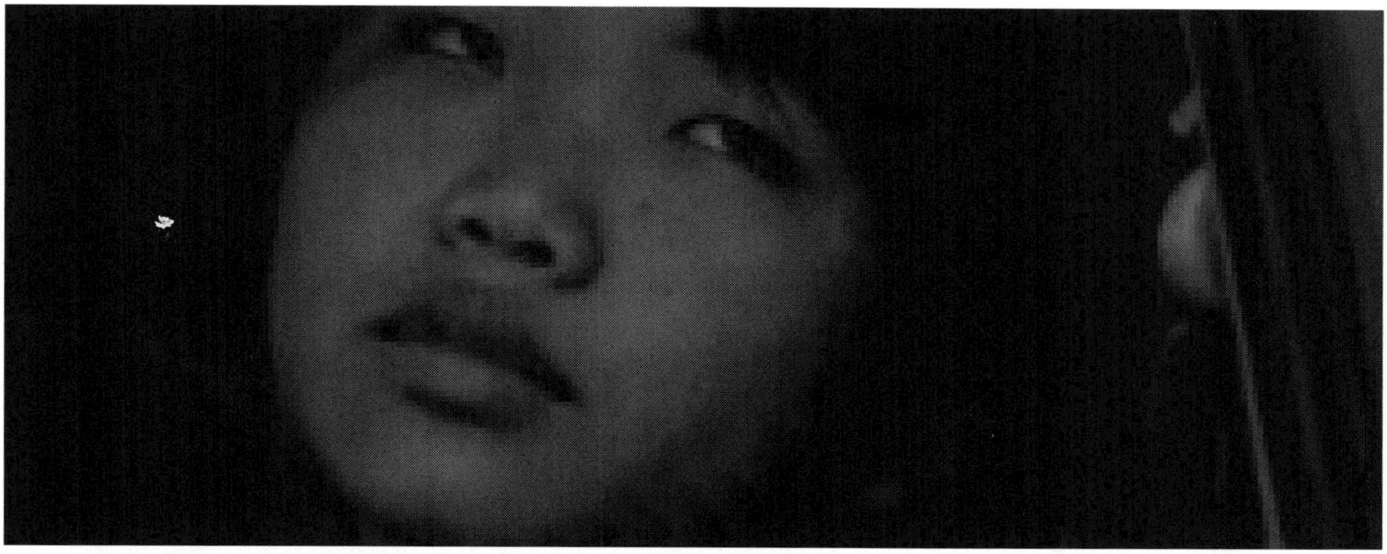

5 16 Y/O MALE, ALTERED MENTAL STATUS, POSSIBLE STROKE

DISPATCH

Location: Suburban home

Type of situation:AMS, possible stroke

Number of patients: 1

Hazards: No hazards

OBJECTIVES

1. Assessment of the patient
2. Prioritize interventions
3. Recognition of hypoglycemia
4. reat symptomatic hypoglycemia
5. Assess effectiveness of interventions
6 Recognize need for priority transport
7. Demonstrate high performance teamwork

SCENE SIZE-UP	
OVERALL SAFETY	SCENE IS SAFE
MOI / NOI	ALTERED MENTAL STATUS, POSSIBLE STROKE
RESOURCES	ALS RESPONSE
C-SPINE	NO SIGNS OF TRAUMA

DIABETIC EMERGENCY

QUESTIONS

Pause 1

Knowledge 0.26

WHAT SCENE SAFETY CONCERNS DO YOU HAVE FOR THIS CALL?

WHAT ARE POSSIBLE CAUSES OF ALTERED MENTAL STATUS?

Pause 2

Assessment 1.31

WHAT CAN YOU GATHER FROM THIS NEW INFORMATION?

Pause 3

Communication 1.52

HOW WILL YOU RESPOND TO THE PATIENT'S REQUEST TO BE LEFT ALONE?

Pause 4

Assessment 2.01

WHAT DO YOU WANT TO DO FIRST AND WHY?

QUESTIONS

Pause 5

Skill 2.40

DESCRIBE THE STEPS OF USING A GLUCOMETER

Pause 6

Assessment 2.43

WHAT DO THE FINDINGS INDICATE?

Pause 7

Skill 2.55

WHAT WOULD YOU DO NEXT?

WHAT ARE THE CONTRAINDICATIONS FOR ORAL GLUCOSE?

Pause 8

Stroke Scale 3.13

DISCUSS HYPOGLYCEMIA AND ITS EFFECTS ON THE BODY.

Pause 9

Assessment 3.27

WHAT ARE YOUR PRIORITIES IN THE AMBULANCE?

Pause 10

Knowledge 3.59

WHY IS THE PATIENT SHIVERING AND HOW WILL YOU TREAT?

QUESTIONS

Pause 11

Knowledge 4.26

WHAT TYPE OF PUMP IS THE PATIENT REFERRING TO?

WHAT SHOULD BE DONE IN THIS SITUATION?

Pause 12

Knowledge 4.40

UNDER WHAT CONDITIONS WOULD YOU ALLOW THIS PATIENT TO REFUSE TRANSPORT?

Pause 13

Communication 6. 10

WHAT INFORMATION IS IMPORTANT TO CONVEY IN YOUR RADIO REPORT?

PCR

Documentation

WHAT IS IMPORTANT TO DOCUMENT ON THIS PCR?

REFLECTION

WOULD YOU HAVE DONE ANYTHING DIFFERENTLY FROM THE ACTIONS AND DECISIONS SHOWN IN THE VIDEO ?

CRITIQUE THE PERFORMANCE AND EXPLAIN YOUR THOUGHT PROCESS.

EMS PATIENT CARE REPORT (PCR) Scenario:

PATIENT INFORMATION

Name:	Allergies:
Age:	Medications:
Sex:	Past Medical History:
Weight: Kg (lb)	Chief Complaint:

VITAL SIGNS

Time:	BP:	Pulse:	Respiration:	Sao_2:
Time:	BP:	Pulse:	Respiration:	Sao_2:
Time:	BP:	Pulse:	Respiration:	Sao_2:

PHYSICAL / NEUROLOGICAL EXAM

LOC:	Skin:	AB/GI:
Oriented:	HEENT:	Pelvis:
GCS:	Neck:	GU:
Pupils:	Chest:	Posterior :
Sensory/Motor:	Respiratory:	Extremities:
Facial Droop:	Cardiovascular:	Psychiatric:
Speech:	EKG:	GLU:

CHIEF COMPLAINT

HISTORY OF PRESENT ILLNESS

NOTES

EMS PATIENT CARE REPORT (PCR) Scenario:

PATIENT INFORMATION

Name:	Allergies:
Age:	Medications:
Sex:	Past Medical History:
Weight: Kg (lb)	Chief Complaint:

VITAL SIGNS

Time:	BP:	Pulse:	Respiration:	Sao_2:
Time:	BP:	Pulse:	Respiration:	Sao_2:
Time:	BP:	Pulse:	Respiration:	Sao_2:

PHYSICAL / NEUROLOGICAL EXAM

LOC:	Skin:	AB/GI:
Oriented:	HEENT:	Pelvis:
GCS:	Neck:	GU:
Pupils:	Chest:	Posterior :
Sensory/Motor:	Respiratory:	Extremities:
Facial Droop:	Cardiovascular:	Psychiatric:
Speech:	EKG:	GLU:

CHIEF COMPLAINT

HISTORY OF PRESENT ILLNESS

NOTES

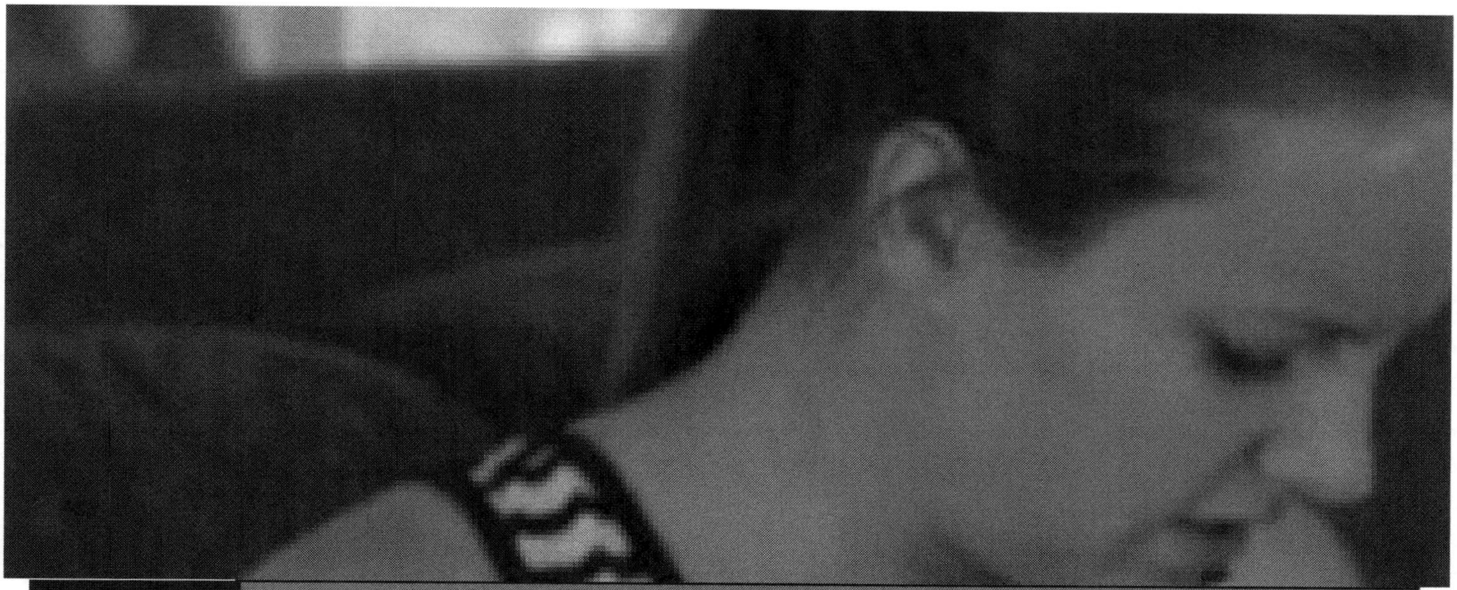

6 24 Y/O FEMALE, IMMINENT BIRTH

DISPATCH
Location: Suburban home
Type of situation: 38 weeks pregnant, water broke, contractions
Number of patients: 2
Hazards: No hazards

OBJECTIVES
1. Assessment of the mother before, during and after birth
2. Recognize imminent birth
3. Assessment of the newborn
4. Understanding of the pathophysiology of birth
5. Prioritization of interventions for uncomplicated delivery of term newborn and placenta
6. Recognize complicated birth situations and appropriate responses
7. Demonstration of effective teamwork

SCENE SIZE-UP	
OVERALL SAFETY	SCENE IS SAFE
MOI / NOI	IMMINENT BIRTH
RESOURCES	BLS RESPONSE
C-SPINE	NO SIGNS OF TRAUMA

NORMAL DELIVERY

QUESTIONS

Pause 1

Knowledge 0.57

WHAT ARE YOUR INITIAL CONCERNS IN RESPONDING TO THIS PATIENT?

Pause 2

Assessment 1.39

HOW WILL YOU ASSESS THE MOTHER TO DETERMINE IF SHE IS READY TO DELIVER?

Pause 3

Assessment 2.44

HOW WILL YOU PERFORM A PHYSICAL EXAMINATION OF THIS PATIENT?

Pause 4

Assessment 3.00

WHAT IS THE SIGNIFICANCE OF CROWNING?

CAN THE MOTHER BE TRANSPORTED TO THE HOSPITAL TO DELIVER?

QUESTIONS

Pause 5

Communication 3.13

HOW WILL YOU INFORM THE MOTHER THAT TRANSPORT IS NOT AN OPTION?

Pause 6

Knowledge 3.39

WHY WAS THE MOTHER PLACED ON THE STRETCHER?

DESCRIBE HOW YOU WOULD POSITION THE MOTHER?

Pause 7

Skill 4.30

DESCRIBE THE STEPS IN MANAGING DELIVERY.

Pause 8

Assessment 5.21

WHAT ARE IMPORTANT ACTIONS ONCE THE BABY HAS DELIVERED?

Pause 9

Skill 5.33

HOW WOULD YOU CUT THE UMBILICAL CORD?

Pause 10

Assessment 6.13

WHAT ASSESSMENT IS NOW NEEDED ON THE MOTHER?

QUESTIONS

Pause 11

Assessment 6.31

DESCRIBE THE USE OF THE APGAR SCALE?

Pause 12

Transport 6.57

HOW SHOULD MOTHER AND CHILD BE TRANSPORTED?

Pause 13

Assessment 7.06

WHAT ARE YOUR ASSESSMENT PRIORITIES DURING TRANSPORT?

Pause 14

Skill 8.06

WHAT IS IMPORTANT IN DELIVERING THE PLACENTA?

REPORT

WHAT INFORMATION IS IMPORTANT TO CONVEY IN YOUR RADIO REPORT?

PCR

In addition to report findings:

REFLECTION

WOULD YOU HAVE DONE ANYTHING DIFFERENTLY FROM THE ACTIONS AND DECISIONS SHOWN IN THE VIDEO ?

CRITIQUE THE PERFORMANCE AND EXPLAIN YOUR THOUGHT PROCESS.

EMS PATIENT CARE REPORT (PCR) Scenario:

PATIENT INFORMATION

Name:	Allergies:
Age:	Medications:
Sex:	Past Medical History:
Weight: Kg (lb)	Chief Complaint:

VITAL SIGNS

Time:	BP:	Pulse:	Respiration:	Sao_2:
Time:	BP:	Pulse:	Respiration:	Sao_2:
Time:	BP:	Pulse:	Respiration:	Sao_2:

PHYSICAL / NEUROLOGICAL EXAM

LOC:	Skin:	AB/GI:
Oriented:	HEENT:	Pelvis:
GCS:	Neck:	GU:
Pupils:	Chest:	Posterior :
Sensory/Motor:	Respiratory:	Extremities:
Facial Droop:	Cardiovascular:	Psychiatric:
Speech:	EKG:	GLU:

CHIEF COMPLAINT

HISTORY OF PRESENT ILLNESS

NOTES

EMS PATIENT CARE REPORT (PCR) Scenario:

PATIENT INFORMATION

Name:
Age:
Sex:
Weight: Kg (lb)

Allergies:
Medications:
Past Medical History:
Chief Complaint:

VITAL SIGNS

Time:	BP:	Pulse:	Respiration:	Sao_2:
Time:	BP:	Pulse:	Respiration:	Sao_2:
Time:	BP:	Pulse:	Respiration:	Sao_2:

PHYSICAL / NEUROLOGICAL EXAM

LOC:
Oriented:
GCS:
Pupils:
Sensory/Motor:
Facial Droop:
Speech:

Skin:
HEENT:
Neck:
Chest:
Respiratory:
Cardiovascular:
EKG:

AB/GI:
Pelvis:
GU:
Posterior :
Extremities:
Psychiatric:
GLU:

CHIEF COMPLAINT

HISTORY OF PRESENT ILLNESS

NOTES

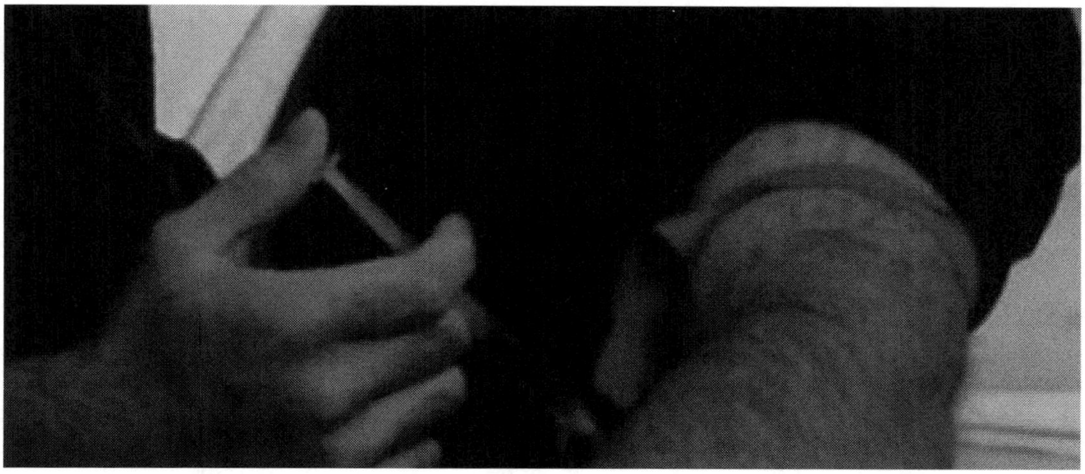

7 UNRESPONSIVE 25 Y/O MALE POSSIBLE OVERDOSE

DISPATCH
Location: Low rent motel room.
Type of situation: Unconscious
Number of patients: 1
Hazards: A syringe and open needle next to patient

OBJECTIVES
1. Discuss Scene Safety considerations for a possible overdose patient
2. Describe the Assessment and Treatment of a patient with a possible overdose
3. Understand the role of Airway Management in the possible overdose patient
4. Prioritize and perform appropriate interventions.
5. Describe the steps in the administration of intranasal medications
6. Demonstrate effective teamwork.

SCENE SIZE-UP	
OVERALL SAFETY	POLICE ARE ON SCENE
MOI / NOI	NARCOTIC OVERDOSE
RESOURCES	ALS RESPONSE
C-SPINE	NO SIGNS OF TRAUMA

OVERDOSE CASE

QUESTIONS

Pause 1

Knowledge 1.01

WHAT SAFETY CONCERNS DO YOU HAVE?

WHAT ARE SOME SIGNS AND SYMPTOMS OF DRUG OVERDOSE?

AFTER SAFETY WHAT ARE YOUR CONCERNS?

Pause 2

Assessment 2.22

WHAT IS YOUR IMPRESSION FROM THE DOOR?

Pause 3

Knowledge 2.40

WHAT ARE YOUR INITIAL PRIORITIES ON SCENE ?

Pause 4

Knowledge 2.49

WHAT DO YOU WANT TO DO FIRST?

QUESTIONS

Pause 5

Knowledge 3.54

WHAT DO THE FINDINGS INDICATE?

WHAT IS YOUR NEXT ACTION? HOW LONG WILL IT TAKE TO TAKE EFFECT?

WHAT IF INTERVENTION DOES NOT WORK?

Pause 6

Skill 4.00

DESCRIBE THE PROCEDURE

Pause 7

Skill 4.25

DESCRIBE ANY OTHER ACTION YOU WOULD PERFORM

WHAT IF THE PATIENT DOES NOT IMPROVE?

ALS 12 LEAD SHOWN

Pause 8

Knowledge 5.41

WHERE SHOULD THIS PATIENT BE TRANSPORTED?

WHAT SHOULD YOU ANTICIPATE?

Pause 9

Assessment 5.57

WHAT ARE YOUR PRIORITIES DURING TRANSPORT?

Pause 10

Communication/ Affect 6.47

CAN THIS PATIENT BE RELEASED? HOW WILL YOU HANDLE?

QUESTIONS

Pause 11

Communication 7.00

WHAT INFORMATION IS IMPORTANT TO CONVEY IN YOUR RADIO REPORT?

PCR

Communication

WHAT IS IMPORTANT TO DOCUMENT ON THIS PCR?

REFLECTION

WOULD YOU HAVE DONE ANYTHING DIFFERENTLY FROM THE ACTIONS AND DECISIONS SHOWN IN THE VIDEO ?

CRITIQUE THE PERFORMANCE AND EXPLAIN YOUR THOUGHT PROCESS.

EMS PATIENT CARE REPORT (PCR) Scenario:

PATIENT INFORMATION

Name:	Allergies:
Age:	Medications:
Sex:	Past Medical History:
Weight: Kg (lb)	Chief Complaint:

VITAL SIGNS

Time:	BP:	Pulse:	Respiration:	Sao_2:
Time:	BP:	Pulse:	Respiration:	Sao_2:
Time:	BP:	Pulse:	Respiration:	Sao_2:

PHYSICAL / NEUROLOGICAL EXAM

LOC:	Skin:	AB/GI:
Oriented:	HEENT:	Pelvis:
GCS:	Neck:	GU:
Pupils:	Chest:	Posterior :
Sensory/Motor:	Respiratory:	Extremities:
Facial Droop:	Cardiovascular:	Psychiatric:
Speech:	EKG:	GLU:

CHIEF COMPLAINT

HISTORY OF PRESENT ILLNESS

NOTES

EMS PATIENT CARE REPORT (PCR) Scenario:

PATIENT INFORMATION

Name:	Allergies:
Age:	Medications:
Sex:	Past Medical History:
Weight: Kg (lb)	Chief Complaint:

VITAL SIGNS

Time:	BP:	Pulse:	Respiration:	Sao_2:
Time:	BP:	Pulse:	Respiration:	Sao_2:
Time:	BP:	Pulse:	Respiration:	Sao_2:

PHYSICAL / NEUROLOGICAL EXAM

LOC:	Skin:	AB/GI:
Oriented:	HEENT:	Pelvis:
GCS:	Neck:	GU:
Pupils:	Chest:	Posterior :
Sensory/Motor:	Respiratory:	Extremities:
Facial Droop:	Cardiovascular:	Psychiatric:
Speech:	EKG:	GLU:

CHIEF COMPLAINT

HISTORY OF PRESENT ILLNESS

NOTES

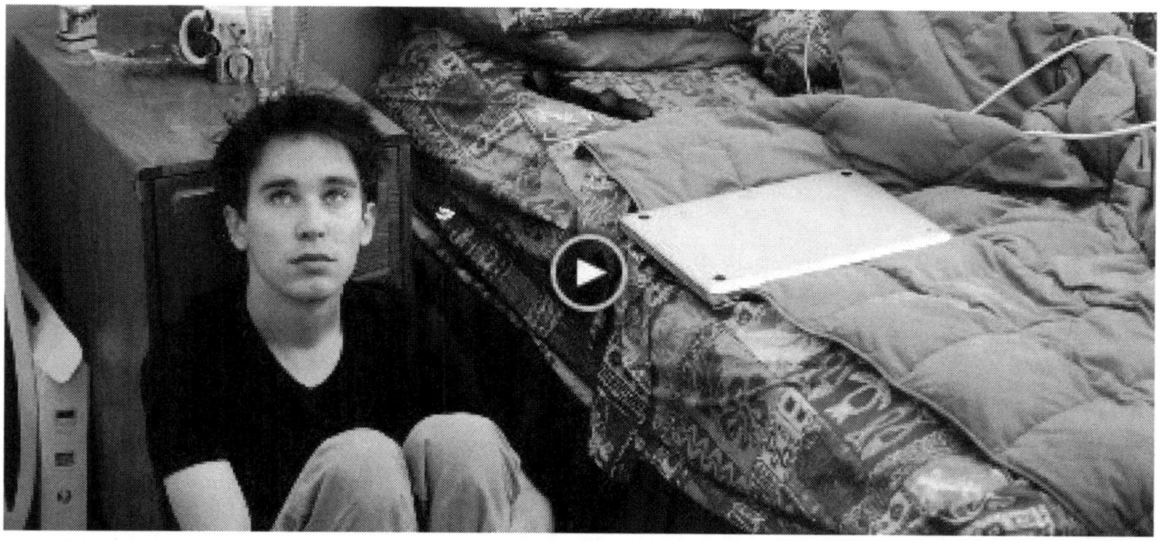

8 24 Y/O MALE, ALTERED MENTAL STATUS

DISPATCH
Location: Suburban home
Type of situation: AMS, possible psychiatric emergency
Number of patients: 1
Hazards: No hazards

OBJECTIVES

1. Scene safety
2. Understanding of the pathophysiology of Mental Illness
3. Prioritization and performance of appropriate interventions
4. Recognition the signs and symptoms of Mental Illness
5. Demonstration of compassion and non-judgmental attitude.
6. Demonstration of effective teamwork

SCENE SIZE-UP	
OVERALL SAFETY	SCENE IS SAFE, PD ON SCENE
MOI / NOI	ALTERED MENTAL STATUS, POSSIBLE PSYCHIATRIC EMERGENCY
RESOURCES	BLS RESPONSE
C-SPINE	NO SIGNS OF TRAUMA

SCHIZOPHRENIA

QUESTIONS

Pause 1

Knowledge 1.01

WHAT SCENE SAFETY CONCERNS DO YOU HAVE FOR THIS CALL?

WHAT ARE POSSIBLE CAUSES OF ALTERED MENTAL STATUS? T

Pause 2

Assessment 1.59

WHAT CAN YOU GATHER FROM THIS NEW INFORMATION?

Pause 3

Assessment 2.20

DESCRIBE THE PATHOPHYSIOLOGY OF SCHIZOPHRENIA

I

Pause 4

Communication 2.27

IS IT SAFE TO LEAVE THE PATIENT WAIT TO SEEK MEDICAL ATTENTION?

QUESTIONS

Pause 5

Communication 2.44

DISCUSS COMMUNICATION STRATEGIES WITH A SCHIZOPHRENIC PATIENT.

Pause 6

Knowledge 3.19

WHAT IS IMPORTANT DURING TRANSPORT?

Pause 7

Skill 3.44

HOW SHOULD THE PROVIDERS RESPOND TO THE PATIENT'S CHANGE?

Pause 8

Knowledge ALS 4.42

WHAT TYPE OF MEDICATION WILL THE MEDIC ADMINiSTER TO THE PATIENT?

Pause 9

Communication 5.42

WHAT INFORMATION IS IMPORTANT TO CONVEY IN YOUR RADIO REPORT?

1. Unit ID, receiving facility, ETA

PCR and REFLECTION

WHAT IS IMPORTANT TO DOCUMENT ON THIS PCR?

DISCUSS THE PROVIDER'S DECISION MAKING ON THIS CALL.

EMS PATIENT CARE REPORT (PCR) Scenario:

PATIENT INFORMATION

Name:	Allergies:
Age:	Medications:
Sex:	Past Medical History:
Weight: Kg (lb)	Chief Complaint:

VITAL SIGNS

Time:	BP:	Pulse:	Respiration:	Sao_2:
Time:	BP:	Pulse:	Respiration:	Sao_2:
Time:	BP:	Pulse:	Respiration:	Sao_2:

PHYSICAL / NEUROLOGICAL EXAM

LOC:	Skin:	AB/GI:
Oriented:	HEENT:	Pelvis:
GCS:	Neck:	GU:
Pupils:	Chest:	Posterior :
Sensory/Motor:	Respiratory:	Extremities:
Facial Droop:	Cardiovascular:	Psychiatric:
Speech:	EKG:	GLU:

CHIEF COMPLAINT

HISTORY OF PRESENT ILLNESS

NOTES

EMS PATIENT CARE REPORT (PCR) Scenario:

PATIENT INFORMATION

Name:	Allergies:
Age:	Medications:
Sex:	Past Medical History:
Weight: Kg (lb)	Chief Complaint:

VITAL SIGNS

Time:	BP:	Pulse:	Respiration:	Sao_2:
Time:	BP:	Pulse:	Respiration:	Sao_2:
Time:	BP:	Pulse:	Respiration:	Sao_2:

PHYSICAL / NEUROLOGICAL EXAM

LOC:	Skin:	AB/GI:
Oriented:	HEENT:	Pelvis:
GCS:	Neck:	GU:
Pupils:	Chest:	Posterior :
Sensory/Motor:	Respiratory:	Extremities:
Facial Droop:	Cardiovascular:	Psychiatric:
Speech:	EKG:	GLU:

CHIEF COMPLAINT

HISTORY OF PRESENT ILLNESS

NOTES

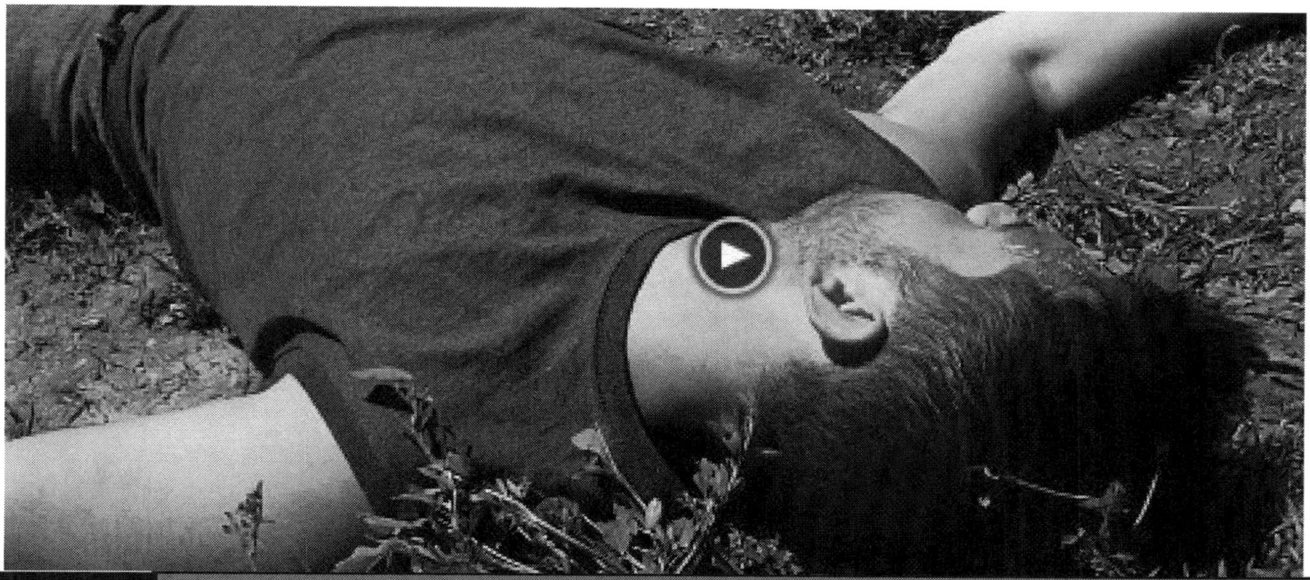

9 21 Y/O MALE, HEAD INJURY AFTER ATV CRASH

DISPATCH
Location: Rural trail
Number of patients: 1
Type of situation:Head injury, ATV crash
Hazards: Unknown
Hospitals: Regional Hospital 20 minutes, Level 1 Trauma 50 minutes

OBJECTIVES

a. Assessment of the patient
b. Prioritize interventions
c. Recognition of head injury
d. Perform correct and timely interventions – airway mngt
e. Appropriate transport decision
f. Demonstrate effective teamwork

SCENE SIZE-UP	
OVERALL SAFETY	UNKNOWN
MOI / NOI	ALTERED MENTAL STATUS, HEAD INJURY AFTER ATV CRASH, EXTENSIVE DAMAGE ATV
RESOURCES	BLS RESPONSE, FD DISPATCHED
C-SPINE	POSSIBLE TRAUMA

HEAD INJURY

QUESTIONS

Pause 1

Knowledge 0.30

WHAT SCENE SAFETY AND LOGISTICS CONCERNS DO YOU HAVE FOR THIS CALL?

WHAT ARE COMMON TYPES OF HEAD INJURY?

Pause 2

Assessment 1.36

WHAT CAN YOU GATHER FROM THIS NEW INFORMATION?

DOES THIS PATIENT MEET THE CRITERIA FOR TRANSPORT TO A TRAUMA CENTER?

Pause 3

Assessment 1.55

WHAT ARE YOUR ASSESSMENT PRIORITIES?

Pause 4

Assessment 2.30

WHAT IS YOUR IMPRESSION OF THE PATIENT BASED ON PRIMARY ASSESSMENT?

QUESTIONS

Pause 5

Knowledge 2.55

WHAT FINDINGS SUPPORTS THE BLEED CONCLUSION? WHAT ADDITIONAL FINDINGS WOULD REINFORCE THIS CONCLUSION?

Pause 6

Knowledge 3.07

HOW POTENTIALLY SERIOUS IS THIS PATIENT AND WHAT ARE YOUR PRIORITIES?

Pause 7

Assessment 3.30

IS THERE ANYTHING SIGNIFICANT ABOUT THE VITALS?

Pause 8

Skill 4.10

IN WHAT SEQUENCE SHOULD STRAPS BE APPLIED?

Pause 9

Assessment 5.17

THE PATIENT IS NOW UNRESPONSIVE.

WHAT IS IMPORTANT TO DOCUMENT WITH THIS PATIENT?

Pause 10

Teamwork 5.28

HOW WOULD YOU HANDLE A JUNIOR TEAM MEMBER OFFERING UNSOLICITED ADVICE?

QUESTIONS

Pause 11

Reassessment and Transport 5.36

WHAT ARE YOUR PRIORITIES IN THE AMBULANCE?

Pause 12

Assessment 6.14

WHAT IS THE SIGNIFICANCE OF CURRENT VITALS AND DILATED PUPILS?

Pause 13

Skill 6.22

DESCRIBE THE PROPER TECHNIQUE FOR VENTILATING THIS PATIENT.

Pause 14

Assessment 7.22

WHAT IS SIGNIFICANT ABOUT CURRENT VITALS?

Pause 15

ALS 7.37

WHY DID THE PARAMEDIC INTUBATE THIS PATIENT?

Pause 16

Communication 10.55

WHAT INFORMATION IS IMPORTANT TO CONVEY IN YOUR HANDOFF REPORT?

QUESTIONS

PCR

Communication

WHAT IS IMPORTANT TO DOCUMENT ON THIS PCR?

REFLECTION

WOULD YOU HAVE DONE ANYTHING DIFFERENTLY FROM THE ACTIONS AND DECISIONS SHOWN IN THE VIDEO ?

CRITIQUE THE PERFORMANCE AND EXPLAIN YOUR THOUGHT PROCESS.

EMS PATIENT CARE REPORT (PCR) Scenario:

PATIENT INFORMATION

Name:	Allergies:
Age:	Medications:
Sex:	Past Medical History:
Weight: Kg (lb)	Chief Complaint:

VITAL SIGNS

Time:	BP:	Pulse:	Respiration:	Sao_2:
Time:	BP:	Pulse:	Respiration:	Sao_2:
Time:	BP:	Pulse:	Respiration:	Sao_2:

PHYSICAL / NEUROLOGICAL EXAM

LOC:	Skin:	AB/GI:
Oriented:	HEENT:	Pelvis:
GCS:	Neck:	GU:
Pupils:	Chest:	Posterior :
Sensory/Motor:	Respiratory:	Extremities:
Facial Droop:	Cardiovascular:	Psychiatric:
Speech:	EKG:	GLU:

CHIEF COMPLAINT

HISTORY OF PRESENT ILLNESS

NOTES

EMS PATIENT CARE REPORT (PCR) Scenario:

PATIENT INFORMATION

Name:	Allergies:
Age:	Medications:
Sex:	Past Medical History:
Weight: Kg (lb)	Chief Complaint:

VITAL SIGNS

Time:	BP:	Pulse:	Respiration:	Sao_2:
Time:	BP:	Pulse:	Respiration:	Sao_2:
Time:	BP:	Pulse:	Respiration:	Sao_2:

PHYSICAL / NEUROLOGICAL EXAM

LOC:	Skin:	AB/GI:
Oriented:	HEENT:	Pelvis:
GCS:	Neck:	GU:
Pupils:	Chest:	Posterior :
Sensory/Motor:	Respiratory:	Extremities:
Facial Droop:	Cardiovascular:	Psychiatric:
Speech:	EKG:	GLU:

CHIEF COMPLAINT

HISTORY OF PRESENT ILLNESS

NOTES

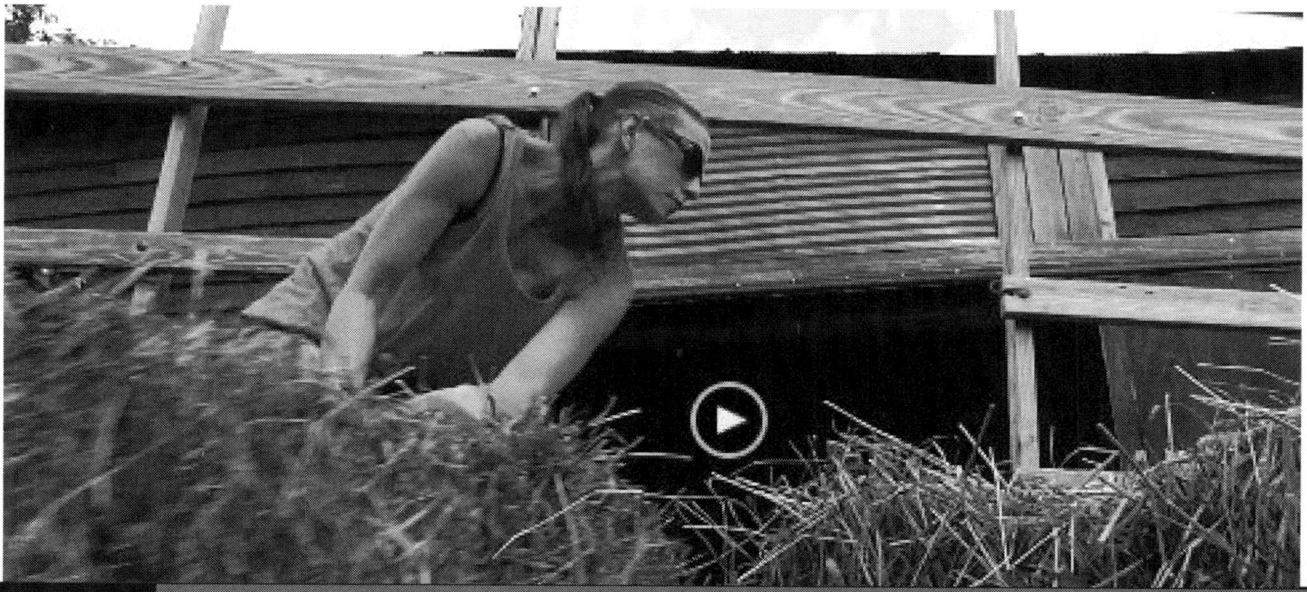

10 36 Y/O FEMALE, OVERHEATED, STOMACH CRAMPS

DISPATCH
Location: Rural farm
Type of situation: Overheated, stomach cramps
Number of patients: 1
Hazards: No hazards, heatwave

OBJECTIVES

1. Assessment of the scene and the patient.
2. Understand the pathophysiology of a heat emergency.
3. Recognize the symptoms of heat cramps, heat exhaustion, and heat stroke.
4. Prioritize and perform appropriate interventions- (cooling the patient, oral fluid replacement)
5. Demonstrate effective teamwork

SCENE SIZE-UP	
OVERALL SAFETY	SCENE IS SAFE
MOI / NOI	OVERHEATED with STOMACH CRAMPS
RESOURCES	BLS RESPONSE
C-SPINE	NO SIGNS OF TRAUMA

HEAT EMERGENCY

QUESTIONS

Pause 1

Knowledge 1.01

WHAT ARE SIGNS AND SYMPTOMS ASSOCIATED WITH HEAT EMERGENCY CONDITIONS?

Pause 2

Assessment 2.08

WHAT ARE ASSESSMENT PRIORITIES WITH THIS PATIENT?

Pause 3

Assessment 2.40

WHAT IS YOUR IMPRESSION OF THIS PATIENT?

Pause 4

Knowledge 3.16

WHAT DO YOU WANT TO DO NEXT AND WHY?

QUESTIONS

Pause 5

Knowledge 4.13

WHAT ARE THE INTERVENTION PRIORITIES FOR HEAT EXHAUSTION COMPARED TO HEAT STROKE?

Pause 6

Communication 4.25

DESCRIBE HOW YOU WOULD UPDATE YOUR NEW COLLEAGUE?

Pause 7

Knowledge 5.29

WHAT FLUIDS SHOULD THIS PATIENT BE GIVEN? ARE THERE ANY CONTRAINDICATIONS?

Pause 8

ALS INTERVENTIONS 5.47

Since the patient cannot drink the ALS providers will quickly start an IV and deliver fluids via that route to rapidly hydrate the patient.

The patient will be placed on the monitor.

Pause 9

Assessment 6.51

WHAT DO THE VITALS INDICATE?

Pause 10

Assessment 7.05

IS ANYTHING CONCERNING IN HER HISTORY?

IS THERE ANY ADDITIONAL INFORMATION YOU'D GATHER FROM THE PATIENT?

QUESTIONS

Pause 11

Communication 7.00

WHAT INFORMATION IS IMPORTANT TO CONVEY IN YOUR RADIO REPORT?

PCR

Communication

WHAT IS IMPORTANT TO DOCUMENT ON THIS PCR?

REFLECTION

WOULD YOU HAVE DONE ANYTHING DIFFERENTLY FROM THE ACTIONS AND DECISIONS SHOWN IN THE VIDEO ?

CRITIQUE THE PERFORMANCE AND EXPLAIN YOUR THOUGHT PROCESS.

EMS PATIENT CARE REPORT (PCR) Scenario:

PATIENT INFORMATION

Name:	Allergies:
Age:	Medications:
Sex:	Past Medical History:
Weight: Kg (lb)	Chief Complaint:

VITAL SIGNS

Time:	BP:	Pulse:	Respiration:	Sao_2:
Time:	BP:	Pulse:	Respiration:	Sao_2:
Time:	BP:	Pulse:	Respiration:	Sao_2:

PHYSICAL / NEUROLOGICAL EXAM

LOC:	Skin:	AB/GI:
Oriented:	HEENT:	Pelvis:
GCS:	Neck:	GU:
Pupils:	Chest:	Posterior :
Sensory/Motor:	Respiratory:	Extremities:
Facial Droop:	Cardiovascular:	Psychiatric:
Speech:	EKG:	GLU:

CHIEF COMPLAINT

HISTORY OF PRESENT ILLNESS

NOTES

EMS PATIENT CARE REPORT (PCR) Scenario:

PATIENT INFORMATION

Name:	Allergies:
Age:	Medications:
Sex:	Past Medical History:
Weight: Kg (lb)	Chief Complaint:

VITAL SIGNS

Time:	BP:	Pulse:	Respiration:	Sao_2:
Time:	BP:	Pulse:	Respiration:	Sao_2:
Time:	BP:	Pulse:	Respiration:	Sao_2:

PHYSICAL / NEUROLOGICAL EXAM

LOC:	Skin:	AB/GI:
Oriented:	HEENT:	Pelvis:
GCS:	Neck:	GU:
Pupils:	Chest:	Posterior :
Sensory/Motor:	Respiratory:	Extremities:
Facial Droop:	Cardiovascular:	Psychiatric:
Speech:	EKG:	GLU:

CHIEF COMPLAINT

HISTORY OF PRESENT ILLNESS

NOTES

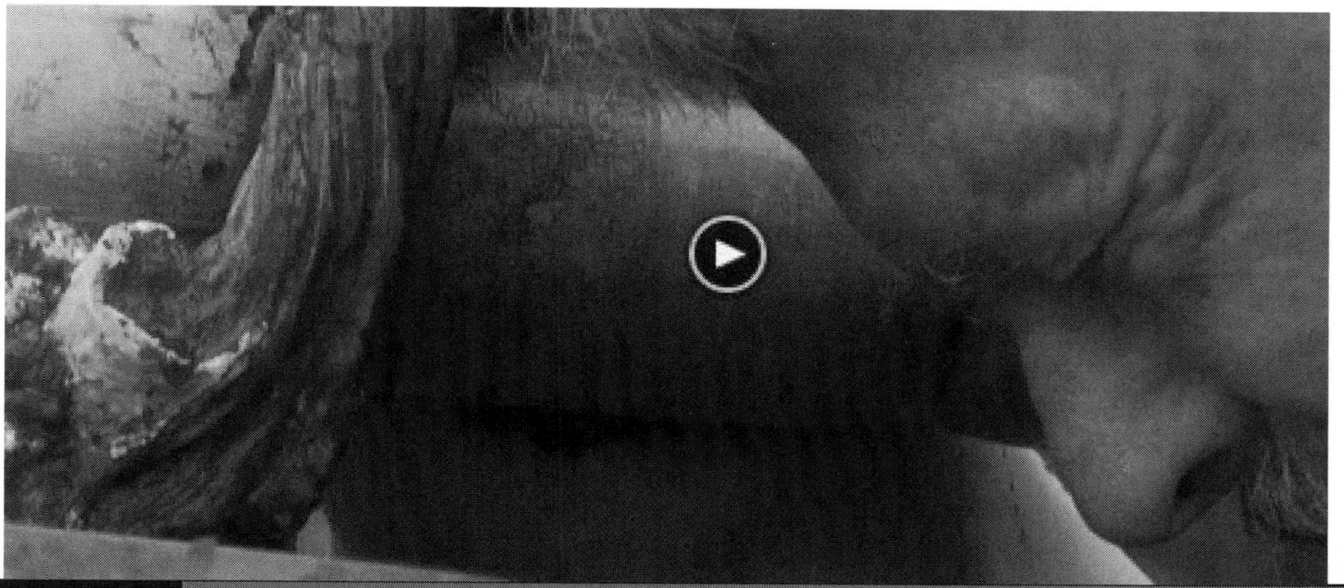

11 55 Y/O MALE, PARTIAL AMPUTATION, EXTREMITY ENTANGLEMENT

DISPATCH
Location: Dairy farm
Type of situation:Partial amputation, trauma
Number of patients: 1
Hazards: Unknown

OBJECTIVES

1. Assessment of the scene and the patient.
2. Recognize need for immediate bleeding control
3. Prioritization and performance of appropriate interventions
4. Recognition of signs and symptoms of shock
5. Recognize need for immediate transport
6. Demonstration of effective teamwork.

SCENE SIZE-UP	
OVERALL SAFETY	FD HAS ALSO BEEN DISPATCHED, TRACTOR STILL RUNNING
MOI / NOI	EXTREMITY ENTANGLEMENT, PARTIAL AMPUTATION, SHOCK
RESOURCES	BLS RESPONSE
C-SPINE	SIGNS OF TRAUMA. PTOs ROTATE AT EXTREMELY HIGH RPM.

PARTIAL AMPUTATION

QUESTIONS

Pause 1

Knowledge 1.05

Background - PTO stands for power Take Off and is a rotating shaft between a tractor and the implement it powers. The PTOs spin at extremely high speeds and a person caught in one can be spun like a rag doll around the shaft resulting in serious injury and often death.

WHAT SCENE SAFETY, SIZE UP AND LOGISTIC CONCERNS DO YOU HAVE FOR THIS CALL.

Pause 2

Assessment 1.48

WHAT INITIAL ACTIONS WILL THE FD TAKE?

Pause 3

Assessment 2.10

WHAT INITIAL ACTIONS SHOULD THE PROVIDERS TAKE?

Pause 4

Communication 2.47

WHAT INFORMATION SHOULD BE OBTAINED / PROVIDED BY THE FIRE DEPARTMENT?

QUESTIONS

Pause 5

Assessment 3.00

WHAT ARE YOUR PRIMARY CONCERNS AS YOU ENTER THE SCENE?

Pause 6

Assessment 3.36

HOW WILL YOU DETERMINE IF SPINAL STABILIZATION IS NEEDED?

Pause 7

Assessment 4.07

WHAT DO THE FINDINGS INDICATE?

Pause 8

Skill 4.19

HOW SHOULD THE WOUNDED EXTREMITY BE TREATED?

WHAT CONCERNS WOULD YOU HAVE WITH A LENGTHY EXTRICATION?

Pause 9

Knowledge 5.00

HOW SHOULD THE PATIENT BE EXTRICATED?

Pause 10

Assessment 6.53

WHAT ARE YOUR PRIORITIES DURING TRANSPORT?

WHERE SHOULD PATIENT BE TRANSPORTED?

QUESTIONS

Pause 11

Skill 7.10

HOW SHOULD THE BLEEDING BE CONTROLLED WITH THE LOSE TOURNIQUET?

Pause 12

Assessment 7.43

DESCRIBE WHAT YOU ARE LOOKING FOR DURING THE DETAILED PHYSICAL EXAM?

Pause 13

Communication 8.41

WHAT INFORMATION IS IMPORTANT TO CONVEY IN YOUR RADIO REPORT?

PCR

Documentation

WHAT IS IMPORTANT TO DOCUMENT ON THIS PCR?

REFLECTION

WOULD YOU HAVE DONE ANYTHING DIFFERENTLY FROM THE ACTIONS AND DECISIONS SHOWN IN THE VIDEO ?

CRITIQUE THE PERFORMANCE AND EXPLAIN YOUR THOUGHT PROCESS.

EMS PATIENT CARE REPORT (PCR) Scenario:

PATIENT INFORMATION

Name:	Allergies:
Age:	Medications:
Sex:	Past Medical History:
Weight: Kg (lb)	Chief Complaint:

VITAL SIGNS

Time:	BP:	Pulse:	Respiration:	Sao_2:
Time:	BP:	Pulse:	Respiration:	Sao_2:
Time:	BP:	Pulse:	Respiration:	Sao_2:

PHYSICAL / NEUROLOGICAL EXAM

LOC:	Skin:	AB/GI:
Oriented:	HEENT:	Pelvis:
GCS:	Neck:	GU:
Pupils:	Chest:	Posterior :
Sensory/Motor:	Respiratory:	Extremities:
Facial Droop:	Cardiovascular:	Psychiatric:
Speech:	EKG:	GLU:

CHIEF COMPLAINT

HISTORY OF PRESENT ILLNESS

NOTES

EMS PATIENT CARE REPORT (PCR) Scenario:

PATIENT INFORMATION

Name:	Allergies:
Age:	Medications:
Sex:	Past Medical History:
Weight: Kg (lb)	Chief Complaint:

VITAL SIGNS

Time:	BP:	Pulse:	Respiration:	Sao_2:
Time:	BP:	Pulse:	Respiration:	Sao_2:
Time:	BP:	Pulse:	Respiration:	Sao_2:

PHYSICAL / NEUROLOGICAL EXAM

LOC:	Skin:	AB/GI:
Oriented:	HEENT:	Pelvis:
GCS:	Neck:	GU:
Pupils:	Chest:	Posterior :
Sensory/Motor:	Respiratory:	Extremities:
Facial Droop:	Cardiovascular:	Psychiatric:
Speech:	EKG:	GLU:

CHIEF COMPLAINT

HISTORY OF PRESENT ILLNESS

NOTES

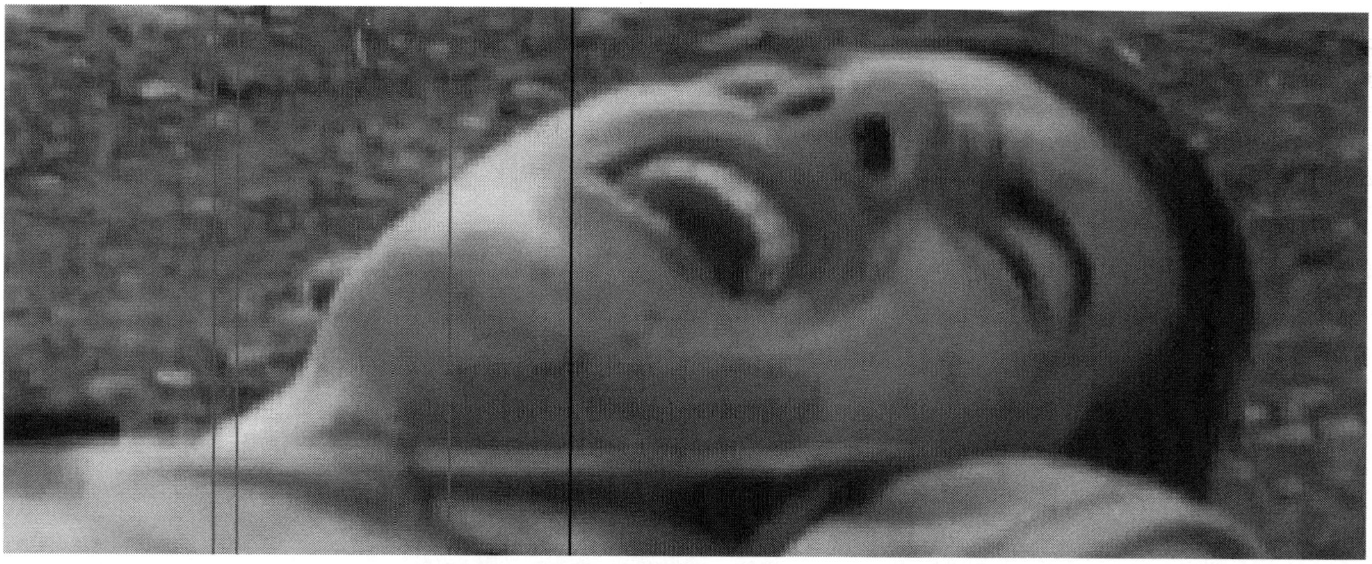

12 21 Y/O MALE, EXTENSIVE UPPER BODY BURNS

DISPATCH

Location: Farm yard

Type of situation: Severe burns

Number of patients: 1

Hazards: Active fire ground

OBJECTIVES

1. Assessment of scene safety.
2. Assessment of the burned patient (BSA)
3. Understand the pathophysiology of burns.
4. Prioritize interventions
5. Perform appropriate interventions.
6. Demonstrate effective teamwork.

SCENE SIZE-UP	
OVERALL SAFETY	ACTIVE FIREGROUND
MOI / NOI	GAS EXPLOSION, EXTENSIVE UPPER BODY BURNS
RESOURCES	BLS RESPONSE
C-SPINE	POSSIBLE TRAUMA

SOFT TISSUE BURN

QUESTIONS

Pause 1

Knowledge 0.31

WHAT SCENE SAFETY and SIZE-UP CONCERNS DO YOU HAVE FOR THIS CALL? WHAT QUESTIONS WILL YOU ASK FIRE FIGHTERS?

WHAT ARE YOUR TREATMENT PRIORITIES LIKELY TO BE AND WHY?

Pause 2

Knowledge 1.37

WHAT IS YOUR GENERAL IMPRESSION?

DISCUSS THE CRITERIA FOR TRANSPORT TO A BURN CENTER AND THIS PATIENT'S NEEDS?

Pause 3

Resources 2.05

WHAT ARE YOUR PRIORITY ASSESSMENTS?

Pause 4

Assessment 2.20

HOW ARE BURNS CLASSIFIED AND HOW IS BSA ASSESSED?

QUESTIONS

Pause 5

Communication 2.55

DISCUSS THE AIRWAY AND BREATHING ASSESSMENT

Pause 6

Stroke Scale 3.13

SHOULD THE WOUNDS BE DRESSED?

Pause 7

Assessment 4.25

WHAT SHORT AND LONG TERM RISKS DOES THIS PATIENT FACE AND HOW CAN THEY BE MANAGED?

Pause 8

ALS Actions 4.55

In order to manage the patient ALS providers will perform a number of interventions including:

* Breathing treatment for wheezes
* 2 IVs for fluid replacement
* Pain management
* Have intubation equipment ready

Pause 9

Knowledge 5.22

WHAT ADDITIONAL ACTIONS ARE NEEDED?

Pause 10

Communication 10 7.03

WHAT INFORMATION IS IMPORTANT TO CONVEY IN YOUR HANDOFF REPORT?

QUESTIONS

PCR

WHAT IS IMPORTANT TO DOCUMENT ON THIS PCR?

REFLECTION

WOULD YOU HAVE DONE ANYTHING DIFFERENTLY FROM THE ACTIONS AND DECISIONS SHOWN IN THE VIDEO ?

CRITIQUE THE PERFORMANCE AND EXPLAIN YOUR THOUGHT PROCESS.

EMS PATIENT CARE REPORT (PCR) Scenario:

PATIENT INFORMATION

Name:	Allergies:
Age:	Medications:
Sex:	Past Medical History:
Weight: Kg (lb)	Chief Complaint:

VITAL SIGNS

Time:	BP:	Pulse:	Respiration:	Sao_2:
Time:	BP:	Pulse:	Respiration:	Sao_2:
Time:	BP:	Pulse:	Respiration:	Sao_2:

PHYSICAL / NEUROLOGICAL EXAM

LOC:	Skin:	AB/GI:
Oriented:	HEENT:	Pelvis:
GCS:	Neck:	GU:
Pupils:	Chest:	Posterior :
Sensory/Motor:	Respiratory:	Extremities:
Facial Droop:	Cardiovascular:	Psychiatric:
Speech:	EKG:	GLU:

CHIEF COMPLAINT

HISTORY OF PRESENT ILLNESS

NOTES

EMS PATIENT CARE REPORT (PCR) Scenario:

PATIENT INFORMATION

Name:	Allergies:
Age:	Medications:
Sex:	Past Medical History:
Weight: Kg (lb)	Chief Complaint:

VITAL SIGNS

Time:	BP:	Pulse:	Respiration:	Sao_2:
Time:	BP:	Pulse:	Respiration:	Sao_2:
Time:	BP:	Pulse:	Respiration:	Sao_2:

PHYSICAL / NEUROLOGICAL EXAM

LOC:	Skin:	AB/GI:
Oriented:	HEENT:	Pelvis:
GCS:	Neck:	GU:
Pupils:	Chest:	Posterior :
Sensory/Motor:	Respiratory:	Extremities:
Facial Droop:	Cardiovascular:	Psychiatric:
Speech:	EKG:	GLU:

CHIEF COMPLAINT

HISTORY OF PRESENT ILLNESS

NOTES

EMS PATIENT CARE REPORT (PCR) Scenario:

PATIENT INFORMATION

Name:	Allergies:
Age:	Medications:
Sex:	Past Medical History:
Weight: Kg (lb)	Chief Complaint:

VITAL SIGNS

Time:	BP:	Pulse:	Respiration:	Sao_2:
Time:	BP:	Pulse:	Respiration:	Sao_2:
Time:	BP:	Pulse:	Respiration:	Sao_2:

PHYSICAL / NEUROLOGICAL EXAM

LOC:	Skin:	AB/GI:
Oriented:	HEENT:	Pelvis:
GCS:	Neck:	GU:
Pupils:	Chest:	Posterior :
Sensory/Motor:	Respiratory:	Extremities:
Facial Droop:	Cardiovascular:	Psychiatric:
Speech:	EKG:	GLU:

CHIEF COMPLAINT

HISTORY OF PRESENT ILLNESS

NOTES

EMS PATIENT CARE REPORT (PCR) Scenario:

PATIENT INFORMATION

Name:	Allergies:
Age:	Medications:
Sex:	Past Medical History:
Weight: Kg (lb)	Chief Complaint:

VITAL SIGNS

Time:	BP:	Pulse:	Respiration:	Sao_2:
Time:	BP:	Pulse:	Respiration:	Sao_2:
Time:	BP:	Pulse:	Respiration:	Sao_2:

PHYSICAL / NEUROLOGICAL EXAM

LOC:	Skin:	AB/GI:
Oriented:	HEENT:	Pelvis:
GCS:	Neck:	GU:
Pupils:	Chest:	Posterior :
Sensory/Motor:	Respiratory:	Extremities:
Facial Droop:	Cardiovascular:	Psychiatric:
Speech:	EKG:	GLU:

CHIEF COMPLAINT

HISTORY OF PRESENT ILLNESS

NOTES

EMS PATIENT CARE REPORT (PCR) Scenario:

PATIENT INFORMATION

Name:	Allergies:
Age:	Medications:
Sex:	Past Medical History:
Weight: Kg (lb)	Chief Complaint:

VITAL SIGNS

Time:	BP:	Pulse:	Respiration:	Sao_2:
Time:	BP:	Pulse:	Respiration:	Sao_2:
Time:	BP:	Pulse:	Respiration:	Sao_2:

PHYSICAL / NEUROLOGICAL EXAM

LOC:	Skin:	AB/GI:
Oriented:	HEENT:	Pelvis:
GCS:	Neck:	GU:
Pupils:	Chest:	Posterior :
Sensory/Motor:	Respiratory:	Extremities:
Facial Droop:	Cardiovascular:	Psychiatric:
Speech:	EKG:	GLU:

CHIEF COMPLAINT

HISTORY OF PRESENT ILLNESS

NOTES

EMS PATIENT CARE REPORT (PCR) Scenario:

PATIENT INFORMATION

Name:	Allergies:
Age:	Medications:
Sex:	Past Medical History:
Weight: Kg (lb)	Chief Complaint:

VITAL SIGNS

Time:	BP:	Pulse:	Respiration:	Sao_2:
Time:	BP:	Pulse:	Respiration:	Sao_2:
Time:	BP:	Pulse:	Respiration:	Sao_2:

PHYSICAL / NEUROLOGICAL EXAM

LOC:	Skin:	AB/GI:
Oriented:	HEENT:	Pelvis:
GCS:	Neck:	GU:
Pupils:	Chest:	Posterior :
Sensory/Motor:	Respiratory:	Extremities:
Facial Droop:	Cardiovascular:	Psychiatric:
Speech:	EKG:	GLU:

CHIEF COMPLAINT

HISTORY OF PRESENT ILLNESS

NOTES

EMS PATIENT CARE REPORT (PCR) Scenario:

PATIENT INFORMATION

Name:	Allergies:
Age:	Medications:
Sex:	Past Medical History:
Weight: Kg (lb)	Chief Complaint:

VITAL SIGNS

Time:	BP:	Pulse:	Respiration:	Sao_2:
Time:	BP:	Pulse:	Respiration:	Sao_2:
Time:	BP:	Pulse:	Respiration:	Sao_2:

PHYSICAL / NEUROLOGICAL EXAM

LOC:	Skin:	AB/GI:
Oriented:	HEENT:	Pelvis:
GCS:	Neck:	GU:
Pupils:	Chest:	Posterior :
Sensory/Motor:	Respiratory:	Extremities:
Facial Droop:	Cardiovascular:	Psychiatric:
Speech:	EKG:	GLU:

CHIEF COMPLAINT

HISTORY OF PRESENT ILLNESS

NOTES

EMS PATIENT CARE REPORT (PCR) Scenario:

PATIENT INFORMATION

Name:	Allergies:
Age:	Medications:
Sex:	Past Medical History:
Weight: Kg (lb)	Chief Complaint:

VITAL SIGNS

Time:	BP:	Pulse:	Respiration:	Sao_2:
Time:	BP:	Pulse:	Respiration:	Sao_2:
Time:	BP:	Pulse:	Respiration:	Sao_2:

PHYSICAL / NEUROLOGICAL EXAM

LOC:	Skin:	AB/GI:
Oriented:	HEENT:	Pelvis:
GCS:	Neck:	GU:
Pupils:	Chest:	Posterior :
Sensory/Motor:	Respiratory:	Extremities:
Facial Droop:	Cardiovascular:	Psychiatric:
Speech:	EKG:	GLU:

CHIEF COMPLAINT

HISTORY OF PRESENT ILLNESS

NOTES

EMS PATIENT CARE REPORT (PCR) Scenario:

PATIENT INFORMATION

Name:	Allergies:
Age:	Medications:
Sex:	Past Medical History:
Weight: Kg (lb)	Chief Complaint:

VITAL SIGNS

Time:	BP:	Pulse:	Respiration:	Sao_2:
Time:	BP:	Pulse:	Respiration:	Sao_2:
Time:	BP:	Pulse:	Respiration:	Sao_2:

PHYSICAL / NEUROLOGICAL EXAM

LOC:	Skin:	AB/GI:
Oriented:	HEENT:	Pelvis:
GCS:	Neck:	GU:
Pupils:	Chest:	Posterior :
Sensory/Motor:	Respiratory:	Extremities:
Facial Droop:	Cardiovascular:	Psychiatric:
Speech:	EKG:	GLU:

CHIEF COMPLAINT

HISTORY OF PRESENT ILLNESS

NOTES

EMS PATIENT CARE REPORT (PCR) Scenario:

PATIENT INFORMATION

Name:	Allergies:
Age:	Medications:
Sex:	Past Medical History:
Weight: Kg (lb)	Chief Complaint:

VITAL SIGNS

Time:	BP:	Pulse:	Respiration:	Sao_2:
Time:	BP:	Pulse:	Respiration:	Sao_2:
Time:	BP:	Pulse:	Respiration:	Sao_2:

PHYSICAL / NEUROLOGICAL EXAM

LOC:	Skin:	AB/GI:
Oriented:	HEENT:	Pelvis:
GCS:	Neck:	GU:
Pupils:	Chest:	Posterior :
Sensory/Motor:	Respiratory:	Extremities:
Facial Droop:	Cardiovascular:	Psychiatric:
Speech:	EKG:	GLU:

CHIEF COMPLAINT

HISTORY OF PRESENT ILLNESS

NOTES

EMS PATIENT CARE REPORT (PCR) Scenario:

PATIENT INFORMATION

Name:	Allergies:
Age:	Medications:
Sex:	Past Medical History:
Weight: Kg (lb)	Chief Complaint:

VITAL SIGNS

Time:	BP:	Pulse:	Respiration:	Sao_2:
Time:	BP:	Pulse:	Respiration:	Sao_2:
Time:	BP:	Pulse:	Respiration:	Sao_2:

PHYSICAL / NEUROLOGICAL EXAM

LOC:	Skin:	AB/GI:
Oriented:	HEENT:	Pelvis:
GCS:	Neck:	GU:
Pupils:	Chest:	Posterior :
Sensory/Motor:	Respiratory:	Extremities:
Facial Droop:	Cardiovascular:	Psychiatric:
Speech:	EKG:	GLU:

CHIEF COMPLAINT

HISTORY OF PRESENT ILLNESS

NOTES

EMS PATIENT CARE REPORT (PCR) Scenario:

PATIENT INFORMATION

Name:	Allergies:
Age:	Medications:
Sex:	Past Medical History:
Weight: Kg (lb)	Chief Complaint:

VITAL SIGNS

Time:	BP:	Pulse:	Respiration:	Sao_2:
Time:	BP:	Pulse:	Respiration:	Sao_2:
Time:	BP:	Pulse:	Respiration:	Sao_2:

PHYSICAL / NEUROLOGICAL EXAM

LOC:	Skin:	AB/GI:
Oriented:	HEENT:	Pelvis:
GCS:	Neck:	GU:
Pupils:	Chest:	Posterior :
Sensory/Motor:	Respiratory:	Extremities:
Facial Droop:	Cardiovascular:	Psychiatric:
Speech:	EKG:	GLU:

CHIEF COMPLAINT

HISTORY OF PRESENT ILLNESS

NOTES

EMS PATIENT CARE REPORT (PCR) Scenario:

PATIENT INFORMATION

Name:	Allergies:
Age:	Medications:
Sex:	Past Medical History:
Weight: Kg (lb)	Chief Complaint:

VITAL SIGNS

Time:	BP:	Pulse:	Respiration:	Sao_2:
Time:	BP:	Pulse:	Respiration:	Sao_2:
Time:	BP:	Pulse:	Respiration:	Sao_2:

PHYSICAL / NEUROLOGICAL EXAM

LOC:	Skin:	AB/GI:
Oriented:	HEENT:	Pelvis:
GCS:	Neck:	GU:
Pupils:	Chest:	Posterior :
Sensory/Motor:	Respiratory:	Extremities:
Facial Droop:	Cardiovascular:	Psychiatric:
Speech:	EKG:	GLU:

CHIEF COMPLAINT

HISTORY OF PRESENT ILLNESS

NOTES

EMS PATIENT CARE REPORT (PCR) Scenario:

PATIENT INFORMATION

Name:
Age:
Sex:
Weight: Kg (lb)

Allergies:
Medications:
Past Medical History:
Chief Complaint:

VITAL SIGNS

Time:	BP:	Pulse:	Respiration:	Sao_2:
Time:	BP:	Pulse:	Respiration:	Sao_2:
Time:	BP:	Pulse:	Respiration:	Sao_2:

PHYSICAL / NEUROLOGICAL EXAM

LOC:	Skin:	AB/GI:
Oriented:	HEENT:	Pelvis:
GCS:	Neck:	GU:
Pupils:	Chest:	Posterior :
Sensory/Motor:	Respiratory:	Extremities:
Facial Droop:	Cardiovascular:	Psychiatric:
Speech:	EKG:	GLU:

CHIEF COMPLAINT

HISTORY OF PRESENT ILLNESS

NOTES

EMS PATIENT CARE REPORT (PCR) Scenario:

PATIENT INFORMATION

Name:	Allergies:
Age:	Medications:
Sex:	Past Medical History:
Weight: Kg (lb)	Chief Complaint:

VITAL SIGNS

Time:	BP:	Pulse:	Respiration:	Sao_2:
Time:	BP:	Pulse:	Respiration:	Sao_2:
Time:	BP:	Pulse:	Respiration:	Sao_2:

PHYSICAL / NEUROLOGICAL EXAM

LOC:	Skin:	AB/GI:
Oriented:	HEENT:	Pelvis:
GCS:	Neck:	GU:
Pupils:	Chest:	Posterior :
Sensory/Motor:	Respiratory:	Extremities:
Facial Droop:	Cardiovascular:	Psychiatric:
Speech:	EKG:	GLU:

CHIEF COMPLAINT

HISTORY OF PRESENT ILLNESS

NOTES

EMS PATIENT CARE REPORT (PCR) Scenario:

PATIENT INFORMATION

Name: Age: Sex: Weight: Kg (lb)	Allergies: Medications: Past Medical History: Chief Complaint:

VITAL SIGNS

Time:	BP:	Pulse:	Respiration:	Sao_2:
Time:	BP:	Pulse:	Respiration:	Sao_2:
Time:	BP:	Pulse:	Respiration:	Sao_2:

PHYSICAL / NEUROLOGICAL EXAM

LOC:	Skin:	AB/GI:
Oriented:	HEENT:	Pelvis:
GCS:	Neck:	GU:
Pupils:	Chest:	Posterior :
Sensory/Motor:	Respiratory:	Extremities:
Facial Droop:	Cardiovascular:	Psychiatric:
Speech:	EKG:	GLU:

CHIEF COMPLAINT

HISTORY OF PRESENT ILLNESS

NOTES

Made in the USA
Monee, IL
05 November 2026

67385932R20079